Wiem Barbaria

Drug intoxication in children

Wiem Barbaria

Drug intoxication in children

A silent scourge

ScienciaScripts

Imprint
Any brand names and product names mentioned in this book are subject to trademark, brand or patent protection and are trademarks or registered trademarks of their respective holders. The use of brand names, product names, common names, trade names, product descriptions etc. even without a particular marking in this work is in no way to be construed to mean that such names may be regarded as unrestricted in respect of trademark and brand protection legislation and could thus be used by anyone.

Cover image: www.ingimage.com

This book is a translation from the original published under ISBN 978-620-6-71118-6.

Publisher:
Sciencia Scripts
is a trademark of
Dodo Books Indian Ocean Ltd. and OmniScriptum S.R.L publishing group

120 High Road, East Finchley, London, N2 9ED, United Kingdom
Str. Armeneasca 28/1, office 1, Chisinau MD-2012, Republic of Moldova, Europe
Printed at: see last page
ISBN: 978-620-7-90467-9

Drug intoxication in children:
Epidemiological, clinical and evolutionary characteristics

I-   Clinical study

Drug poisoning in children is a national and international public health problem. (1). Several Tunisian studies carried out in emergency departments, paediatric intensive care units and general paediatric wards have shown that this type of poisoning is still frequent today, and that its evolution can be fraught with sometimes fatal complications. Mortality is related to age, the type of drug, the nature of the intoxication (single or multiple drug intoxication) and the dose ingested.

Although prevention is the best treatment for drug intoxication, prevention strategies in our country do not appear to be sufficient today to reduce the frequency of these intoxications.

In this study, we propose to describe the epidemiological, clinical and evolutionary characteristics of drug intoxication in children in a general paediatric ward in the governorate of Bizerte.

Methods:

We conducted a retrospective descriptive study of the records of children hospitalized for drug intoxication in the pediatrics department of the Habib Bougatfa Hospital in Bizerte over a 3-year period (January 1, 2019 to December 31, 2021). We would like to point out that any child consulting us for drug intoxication is systematically hospitalized in our department, whatever the nature of the drug, the supposed dose ingested and the child's symptomatology.

Results:

We enrolled 57 children during the study period. Overall incidence was 1.5%. The highest incidence rate was observed in the year 2020 (1.23%) (Figure 1).

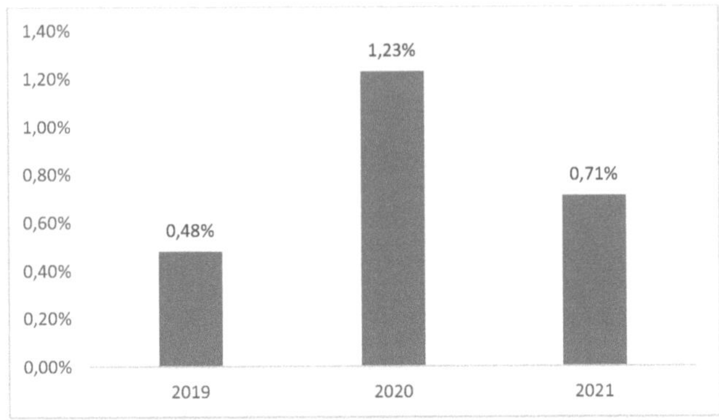

Figure 1: Incidence rates by year

The sex ratio (M/F) was 0.96. The mean age of hospitalized children was 4 years, with extremes ranging from 7 days to 14 years. The majority of children were infants under 3 years of age (69%). Older children and newborns were involved in 28% and 2% respectively. The child hospitalized was the youngest in the family in 44% of cases. Poisoning was accidental in 80% of cases. The drug was administered to the child by mistake in 31.6% of cases. Poisoning occurred in the morning before midday in 62.5% of cases. The most frequent month of poisoning was June (15.8%), and the most frequent season was spring (34%) (Table1).

Table 1: Breakdown of intoxications by month

Month	January	February	March	April	May	June	July	August	September	October	November	December
N	2	5	8	4	7	9	5	4	1	2	6	4
%	3,6	8,7	14	7	12,3	15,8	8,7	7	1,8	3,6	10,5	7

The drug was in the child's diet in 31.6% of cases. A chronic parental pathology was found in 45.5% of children. Neurological pathologies were the most frequent (Table 2).

Table II: Parental pathology of poisoned children

	Maternal pathology	Paternal pathology	Total
Neurological pathology	N=4 7%	N=5 8,8%	N=9 15,8%
Dysthyroidism	N=3 5,2%	N=0	N=3 5,2%
Diabetes	N=2 3,5%	N=2 3,5%	N=4 7%
Hypertension	N=2 3,5%	N=2 3,5%	N=4 7%
Asthma	0	N=2 3,5%	N=2 3,5%
Other	N=3 5,2%	N=1 1,8%	N=4 7%

The average time between intoxication and consultation was 10 hours. Induced vomiting and milk ingestion concerned 15% of children. The most frequently incriminated drugs were neuroleptics (19%), beta2 mimetics (6%) and paracetamol (5%) (Figure 2).

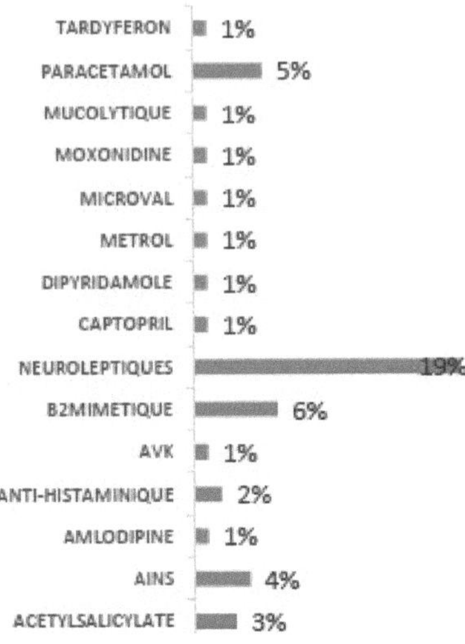

Figure 2: Drugs implicated in pediatric intoxications

Poly-drug intoxication occurred in 11% of cases. The majority of children were asymptomatic on admission. Liver failure was found in 7% of children. Heart and kidney failure were noted in 1.7% of cases. Gastric lavage was performed in 12.3% of children. A specific antidote was administered in 5.2% of children. The average hospital stay was 2 days, with extremes ranging from 1 to 17 days. The outcome was favorable in 87.5% of children. Transfer to intensive care was indicated in 3.5% of children, and death was noted in 28% of cases. Parents discharged their child from our department against medical advice in 10.5% of cases.

Discussion:

Accidental or deliberate drug intoxication in the paediatric population is a real scourge in many countries around the world, and a frequent cause of admission to emergency departments and intensive care units. (2).

In our study, the overall incidence of drug intoxication was 1.5%, but we have no idea of the incidence on a national scale, as there is no register of all cases of drug intoxication in children.

The highest incidence was observed in the year 2020 during the containment period due to the covid 19 pandemic. This finding was also reported in the Raffee et al. study, comparing the incidence of drug poisoning between the years 2019 and 2020. The explanation put forward for this observation was that families stockpiled drugs in anticipation of shortages, alongside a stay-at-home policy; children spent more time at home, increasing their accidental exposure to these drugs (3).

The average age of hospitalized children was 4 years, with extremes ranging from 7 days to 14 years. In a French study, the distribution of drug intoxications was described according to two peaks of frequency: 3 and 14 years of age (4).

In the majority of cases, drug intoxication was accidental (80%) in our study, whereas it was unintentional in only 37% of cases in the study by Molimard et al. (5) .

In our work, the season with the highest rate of drug intoxication was spring, whereas it was winter according to Sinno-Tellier et al. (6)

The drugs incriminated in drug intoxications varied from one study to another, but we note the recurrence of drugs acting: on the nervous system: psychotropic drugs (37%)(5)on the cardiovascular system (20%)(6) and analgesics/anti-inflammatories (41%)(5).

In a Moroccan study, the clinical picture was dominated by neurological signs: disturbed consciousness, behavioral disturbance and convulsion. In the majority of cases, treatment was symptomatic. Detoxification measures were reported in 10% of cases.(7).

Only 0.5% to 2% of drug intoxications require treatment in a pediatric intensive care unit. Mortality is low and increases with age, according to a French study (4).

Pediatric drug poisoning is common, but preventable. Awareness-raising campaigns for parents via the media and social networks are therefore essential.

Toxicological research must be systematic, to document the type of intoxication and initiate specific treatment if possible. We therefore propose to base a poison control center in the region to facilitate the use of toxicological research.

Conclusion:

Drug poisoning in children is a real public health problem. The natural curiosity of young children, combined with the fact that medicines are sometimes too easily accessible, creates a major risk of accidents in the home. Given this situation, vigilance and prevention are essential. Parents and responsible adults must adopt strict safety measures to limit access to medicines.

References:

1. Sahin S, Bora Carman K, Dinleyici EC. Acute Poisoning in Children; Data of a Pediatric Emergency Unit. Iran J Pediatr. Dec 2011;21(4):479-84.

2 Attazagharti N, Soulaymani A, Ouami L, Mokhtari A, Soulaymani BR. Drug intoxications and risk factors influencing patient outcome. Antropo. 2009;(19):33-9.

3. Raffee L, Daradkeh HM, Alawneh K, Al-Fwadleh AI, Darweesh M, Hammad NH, et al. Impact of COVID-19 lockdown on the incidence and patterns of toxic exposures and poisoning in Jordan: a retrospective descriptive study. BMJ Open. 9 Dec 2021;11(12):e053028.

4. Brissaud O, Chevret L, Claudet I. Severe intoxication by drugs and/or illicit substances admitted to intensive care: pediatric specificities. Réanimation. Oct 2006;15(5):405-11.

5. Molimard J, Blanc I, Létinier L, Titier K, Bouchet S, Pillet P, et al. Epidemiology of intoxications by drugs or psychoactive substances in pediatrics: retrospective study from 2013 to 2018 at Bordeaux University Hospital. Toxicol Anal Clin. March 1, 2021;33(1):7.

6. Sinno-Tellier S, Evrard M, Nardon A, Boels D, Langrand J, Azzouz R, et al. Pediatric accidental poisonings recorded by poison centers from 2014 to 2020. Toxicol Anal Clin. 1 Oct 2023;35(3, Supplement):S82-3.

7. Znaiber M, Soufi L, Salimi S, Dehbi F. P-173 - Drug intoxications in children: about 76 cases. Arch Pediatr. 2015;5 Supplement 1(22):276.

Colchicine intoxication: a special situation in children

Introduction:

Colchicine is a highly toxic tricyclic alkaloid, originally extracted from colchicummainly the autumn colchicum.

Colchicine's anti-inflammatory effect was initially used to prevent or treat gout attacks. Today, it is also approved for the treatment of Mediterranean fever and Behçet's disease. Colchicine is also effective in the management of certain forms of pericarditis. (1) (2) (3)

Described in literature for centuries, colchicine, considered one of the oldest drugs in the pharmacopoeia, is known both as a poison and as a medicine, due to its mechanism of action. In fact, it blocks cell division by inhibiting microtubule polymerization, thus blocking cells in metaphase, and this is at the root of its toxicity. (3) (4)

Digestive signs (nausea, diarrhea, vomiting) are the first to appear in the event of overdose. This is followed by life-threatening polyvisceral damage, as there is no specific antidote.(3) (5)

Very few cases of colchicine intoxication have been reported in the literature. The types of intoxication reported are essentially voluntary and suicidal in adults and adolescents. A few cases of accidental intoxication due to dosage errors have also been reported.

We report the observation of severe voluntary colchicine intoxication in a 13-year-old girl with a favorable outcome.

The objectives of our work are:

1- Analyze the clinical, therapeutic and evolutionary profile of a pediatric case of severe colchicine intoxication.

2- Literature review of the diagnostic, therapeutic and evolutionary aspects of colchicine intoxication.

Observation

Child H.K, 13 years old, admitted through the emergency department for management of abdominal trauma.

- Family **history**:

    - Mother treated for Behçet's disease on colchicine.

- **Personal history**:

    - No particular pathological history.

    - In seventh grade with average performance.

    - No known psychiatric disorders.

- **History of the disease:**

    On the day of admission, following a dizzy spell, the patient suffered a fall from the stairs at home, with abdominal reception. She presented 5 hours later with vomiting and abdominal pain, predominantly epigastric, in a febrile context. An abdomino-pelvic CT scan requested by a free-lance physician revealed an effusion slide in the Douglas. The patient was referred to the Habib Bougatfa University Hospital in Bizerte for emergency care.

- **Initial emergency examination:** General condition altered with fever of 38.2°. Abdominal examination revealed tenderness in the right hypochondrium and epigastrium. The patient was conscious and cooperative, with a Glasgow score of 15/15. Hemodynamically, she had a hypoarterial pressure of 80/60 mmHg, tachycardia at 124 bpm, cold extremities and mottling. Her respiratory status was stable.

- **Immediate course of action:**

5-1- Hospitalization in a surgical intensive care unit

5-2- Hemodynamic disorders corrected with 20mL/kg saline vascular filling.

5-3- Hemodynamic support with norepinephrine 0.1mg/kg/min and dobutamine 10 µg/kg/min by electric syringe via central venous catheter.

5-4- Initial biological workup:

- Hemoglobin normal at 12g/dL, white blood cells at 10,300 el/mm^3 and thrombocytopenia at 117,000 el/mm^3 .

- Renal insufficiency with urea at 0.87 µmol/l, creatinine at 229 µmol/L, hyponatremia at 125mmol/L and normal kalemia.

- Hepatic cytolysis with ALT at 2 times normal and ASAT at 13 times normal associated with hepatocellular failure (TP=51%). Alkaline phosphatase was elevated to 2 times normal (1815 IU/L).

- Blood gases: respiratory alkalosis with pH 7.49; PCO2=27.2 mmHg; HCO3-= 20.3 mmHg.

- Lipasemia: normal at 54 IU/L

- Hypersensitive troponin assay: elevated to 6721 pg/L.

- Creatine phosphatase kinase and lactate dehydrogenase assays elevated to 20580 and 4242 IU/mL respectively.

- Inflammatory syndrome with CRP elevated to 337.12 mg/L

- Blood culture series

- Cytobacteriological examination of urine: direct examination: 1000 el/ml

- PCR COVID: negative

- COVID serology: in progress

5-5- Radiological check-up:

- Chest X-ray: no abnormalities.

- Electrocardiogram: Normal

- Abdominal-pelvic CT scan after 12 hours of trauma: No abnormalities, no effusion, no deep lesions.

6- **All in all:**

Patient aged 13, with no notable pathological history, victim of a fall from the stairs at home with abdominal trauma following vertigo.

Initial examination revealed abdominal pain, altered general condition with fever and poor hemodynamics.

Biological tests showed normal hemoglobin levels, thrombocytopenia, hepatic cytolysis with hepatocellular insufficiency, renal failure, elevated muscle enzymes and troponins, and a biological inflammatory syndrome.

Abdominopelvic CT initially showed a small effusion in the Douglas, which was controlled at H12 post-trauma and returned to normal.

Given this clinico-biological picture, internal haemorrhage was ruled out and the suspected diagnoses were:

1- Sepsis with septic shock and multi-visceral failure.

2- A multi-systemic inflammatory syndrome post COVID.

3- An outbreak of familial Mediterranean fever.

7- **<u>Initial care:</u>**

- The patient was put on systemic probabilistic antibiotics: Cefotaxime: 200mg/kg/D and Gentamicin 5mg/kg/D.

   - Intravenous immunoglobulin 1g/kg.

   - Bolus methylprednisolone 10 mg/kg/d for 3 days, then 2mg/kg/d.

   - Aspegic 5mg/kg (anti-platelet aggregation dose).

   - Restriction of water intake to 800 mL/m^2 body surface area (due to hyponatremia and suspected inappropriate secretion of antidiuretic hormone)

   - Vitamin K 10 mg/d for 3 days.

8 - Immediate evolution: (from D0 to D7)

8-1-Overall:

- General condition and fever persist for 5 days.

<u>8-2-</u> Infection:

- Negative blood cultures after 72 hours.

- CRP checked at 121 and then 71mg/L on D5 and D6 respectively.

- COVID serology: IgM and IgG negative.

- ECBU culture negative.

→ Antibiotic therapy stopped after 3 days.

<u>8-3- Hemodynamics</u>:

- Stabilization of hemodynamic status with vasoactive drugs.

- Echocardiography at day 4: normal: good overall myocardial function, no pericardial effusion.

→ Noradrenaline stopped on day 6 of hospitalization.

<u>8-4- Visceral</u>:

- Persistent renal failure.

- Improvement in troponin, muscle and liver enzyme assays (Table 1).

<u>8-5- Hematology</u>:

- Persistent and progressively worsening thrombocytopenia (Table 1).

<u>8-6- Electrolytically:</u>

- Normalization of natremia at day 5.

→ Adjust electrolyte intake to $1.5L/m^2$ /D by intravenous infusion.

<u>8-7- Neurological: After</u> 5 days in hospital, the patient became agitated, with visual and auditory hallucinations. Glasgow score was 10/15.

<u>8-8- Skin:</u> appearance of cheilitis and perioral vesicular lesions on day 5 (figure 1).

The diagnosis of herpetic encephalitis was evoked. Lumbar puncture could not be performed because of severe thrombocytopenia ($15,000/mm^3$). Cerebral CT scan was without abnormalities. The electroencephalogram was not performed.

→ The patient was transfused with two platelets and put on anti-viral treatment: intravenous Acyclovir.

9-Further developments: (From D7)

9-1- <u>On a general level:</u>

- Lasting apyrexia and partial improvement in general condition.

9-2- Neurological:

- Persistence of visual hallucinations and fluctuating consciousness after 2 days of anti-viral treatment.

9-3- Hepatically:

- reduction in cytolysis and normalization of TP (Table 1).

9-4-   <u>Renal</u>:

- Normalization of renal function.

- Hypokalemia confirmed at 2.82mmol/L

→ Intravenous correction of hypokalemia.

Given the clinico-biological evolution, the absence of arguments in favor of bacterial infection and the evolution of the neurological state under anti-viral treatment, we evoked the diagnosis of drug intoxication, notably colchicine.

On our request to check the mother's colchicine tablets (treated for Behçet's disease), it was indeed reported that four tablets containing 40 colchicine tablets were found empty at home.

The patient's blood colchicine level came back very high at 9 mg/ml. The supposed dose ingested by the patient was 1 mg/kg/d.

→ The diagnosis of acute severe colchicine intoxication was retained and confirmed by colchicinemia levels, the clinico-biological evolution and the appearance of progressive frontal alopecia at D10 (figure 2).

Acyclovir was stopped at D7. Neurological status improved progressively over 13 days. Kalemia was corrected at day 12.

During the child psychiatric interview, the patient declared that she had ingested 40 colchicine tablets with suicidal intent. She was discharged at D 17 with additional child psychiatric follow-up.

Figure 1: Erythematous lips with vesicular lesions (cheilitis)

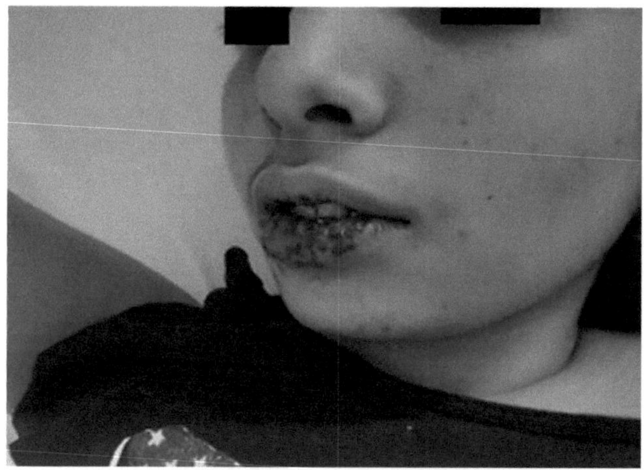

Figure 2: Frontal alopecia

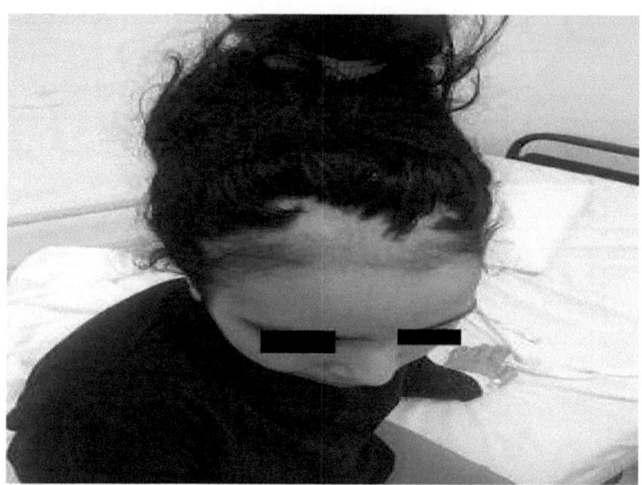

Table 1: Kinetics of biological parameters.

Hospital check-up	J1	J4	J5	J6	J8	J10	J12
GB (/µL)	10300	2900	6700	17200	32750	-	19300
HB (g/dl)	12,5	11,5	10,7	10,4	8,9	-	8,2
VGM (µm3)	87	87	87	86	90	-	96
TCMH (pg)	30,1	30,3	31,3	30,1	28,3	-	32,1
Plq (/µL)	117000	14000	77000	96000	282000	-	311000
CRP (mg/L)	337,12	-	121,69	73,58	22,45	-	6,39
Urea(g/L)/ creat(µmol/L)	0,87/ 229	0,77/ 59	0,95/ 55	0,7/ 38	0,7/ 82	-	0,21/ 51
Na+/K+ (mmol/L)	125,2/ 4,25	129,3/ 4,82	137,9/ 4,8	143,1/ 4,16	141,9/ 2,82	144,4/ 2,68	140,6/ 3,78
AST (U/L)	544	495	215	122	78	-	42
ALAT (U/L)	84	209	182	150	108	-	53
G-GT	-	130	202	262	207	-	-
PAL	1815	208	181	183	-	-	-
TP	51,8	100	-	85	57,3	-	82,3
Fibrinemia (g/L)	3,34	-	-		1,9	-	-
CPK (U/L)	20580	-	2535	-	-	-	390
LDH (U/L)	4242	-	1101	-	-	-	561
Troponins (pg/ml)	6721,6	1255,8	-	-	-	-	-
Albuminemia	-	-	-	-	28,9	-	23,9
Calcemia (corrected calcemia)	-	1,62	-	1,85	1,82 (2.09)	-	1,76 (2.16)
Amylasemia	-	-	122	122	-	-	-
Blood gas:	-	-	pH=7.49 PCO2=27.2 PaO2=80.0 HCO3-=20.3 SaO2=96.9 %	pH=7.48 PCO2=25.7 PaO2=133 HCO3-=21.5 SaO2=99.3%	pH=7.51 PCO2=24.9 PaO2=77 HCO3- =19.8 SaO2=96.8	pH=7.45 PCO2=26.7 PaO2=81 HCO3-=20 SaO2=96.6	pH=7.51 PCO2=24.9 PaO2=77 HCO3-=19.8 SaO2=96.8

DISCUSSION

We report the observation of voluntary colchicine intoxication with suicidal intent in a 13-year-old adolescent girl. The initial clinico-biological picture was not very specific and the intoxication was not announced at the beginning of the treatment, which led to an erroneous diagnosis. On the other hand, adequate management of the various organ failures, even in the absence of a precise etiological diagnosis, led to a favorable outcome. There is no antidote to colchicine. Treatment was symptomatic only.

1- Study highlights:

This is a serious case of colchicine intoxication, rarely reported in the literature. To our knowledge, this is the first case reported in Tunisia.

Our treatment resulted in a favorable outcome despite the parents' failure to report the poisoning.

2- Weaknesses of the study:

We have reported a single observation mono-centrically.

1. Drug characteristics:

1.1 Pharmacokinetics:

For many years, the pharmacokinetics of colchicine and its metabolic destination have remained unknown. Recently, however, these parameters have been defined by the determination of colchicine plasma concentrations using radioimmunological techniques. Two proteins play a major role in colchicine pharmacokinetics: tubulin, the specific intracellular receptor for colchicine, which determines its elimination half-life in the blood, and P-glycoprotein, the cellular detoxification pump that regulates tissue distribution and biliary and renal elimination. (1)

1.1.1. Absorption and bioavailability

When administered orally, colchicine is highly lipophilic and rapidly absorbed from the gastrointestinal tract. However, the fraction of the dose absorbed can vary greatly from one individual to another. Several studies have shown the appearance of a plasma peak between 30 and 90 minutes after ingestion of a single dose of 1mg of colchicine. (6) (7)

The study carried out by Rochdi et al showed great variability in bioavailability, ranging from 24 to 88%, with an average of 45%. (8)

1.1.2. Distribution:

Once absorbed, colchicine is rapidly distributed to all tissues. At therapeutic doses, the volume of distribution is between 7 and 10 L/kg, much higher than the volume of the extracellular space. It can reach up to 21 L/kg in the event of overdose. This volume of distribution is one of the reasons why hemodialysis is ineffective in cases of intoxication. The distribution half-life of colchicine is between 1 and 2.7 hours.(1) Approximately 50% of circulating colchicine is non saturably bound to plasma proteins. Protein binding is mainly to human albumin (40%). (1)

A study by Amoura et al in 1993 (9) demonstrated colchicine's ability to cross the placental barrier, particularly during chronic treatment. Colchicine also passes into milk. Colchicine is still capable of crossing the blood-brain barrier, leading to accumulation in the tubulin-rich brain. The major therapeutic risk in terms of distribution lies mainly in the potential risk of P-gp saturation. This risk is particularly relevant when co-prescribing.

1.1.3. Metabolism and elimination:

Colchicine is metabolized in the liver parenchyma by the cytochrome P-450 pathway, and more specifically by the CYP-3A4 isoform. The latter is located mainly in the intestine and liver, and is essential for the biotransformation of colchicine, which undergoes oxidative demethylation.

Several inhibitors or competitors can modulate P-gp activity, resulting in intracellular accumulation of the drug and a concomitant increase in its pharmacological or toxic activity.

The kidneys also play a role in colchicine clearance. Renal elimination represents 5-20% of total body clearance (depending on the animal species). Renal clearance of colchicine in healthy subjects is of the order of 4 L/h, representing only 10% of total clearance.(10)

The complex pharmacokinetics of colchicine may explain many of the problems encountered by patients undergoing treatment: (11)

¬ Individual variability in colchicine metabolism efficiency, (12)

¬ Reduced elimination in subjects with impaired hepatic and/or renal function,

¬ Drug interactions (macrolides, pristinamycin, statins, etc.) modulating CYP-3A4 or P-gp activity.

2.a.4. Half-life:

The elimination half-life of colchicine, after ingestion of an oral dose, varies between 14 and 30 hours in healthy individuals. (7) (8)

2.b. pharmacodynamics and mechanism of action:

2.b.1.anti-mitotic effect:

Colchicine binds ubiquitously to free tubulins, the proteins that make up microtubules. These microtubules play a key role in cell division. During mitosis, they appear around centrioles, forming the mitotic spindle.

Colchicine's anti-mitotic action consists in its binding to tubulin, which inhibits polymerization of the main constituents of microtubules, thus stopping their elongation and interrupting cell proliferation by blocking the cell at the metaphase stage.(13)

2.b.2 Anti-inflammatory effect:

By inhibiting tubulin site-congestion polymerization, colchicine disrupts other cellular functions involving microtubules, such as cell transport (including granulocytes and monocytes), cell shape maintenance, phagocytosis, intracellular vesicular migration, histamine granule release from mast cells, and cytokine and chemokine secretion. (1)

Colchicine is a fully-fledged anti-inflammatory agent. It slows the influx of leukocytes into the inflammatory zone during an inflammatory reaction, and reduces their adhesion to endothelial cells by modulating the expression of adhesion molecules (E-selectin) and stimulating the expression of L-selectins by leukocytes, thus preventing their recruitment.(14) It also inhibits polynuclear and monocyte chemotaxis and adhesiveness. Phagocytosis is also impaired by inhibition of lysosomal degranulation.

Colchicine also acts on TNFα (tumor necrosis factor α), a mediator of inflammation and a player in chemotaxis, by inhibiting its release during inflammatory episodes by macrophages, thus preventing it from exerting its role in leukocyte recruitment. (1) (15)

2.b.3. Disruption of ion flow:

Once bound to tubulin, colchicine alters the balance of ionic flows. It has an effect on the transmembrane movement of calcium and certain amino acids involved in DNA synthesis. (10) (16)

2.b.4. Other actions of colchicine:

• Colchicine and platelets: Colchicine alters calcium fluxes, reducing platelet aggregation and secretion. (17)

• Colchicine and nerve cells: Colchicine inhibits axonal transport, modifies synapse morphology and inhibits neurotransmission. It can therefore cause axonal neuropathy or necrosis of certain nerve cells. (17)

• Colchicine and endocrine cells: by altering the transfer and exocytosis of intracytoplasmic secretory vesicles, colchicine inhibits the secretion of several hormones, including insulin, thyroid iodine compounds and parathyroid hormone.

• Colchicine and collagen: Colchicine has an anti-fibrosing action, reducing fibrinogen and collagen synthesis. It also promotes collagen degradation by stimulating collagenase synthesis and activity.

. An extended study involving 19 patients described azoospermia in one subject and a deficit in the sperm penetration test in three others, with reversibility of these effects observed on discontinuation of treatment. (18)

2.c. Toxicological analysis:

The therapeutic zone is close to the toxic zone, which explains why colchicine is classified as a drug with a narrow therapeutic margin.

The recommended therapeutic dosage of colchicine according to the patient's age is:(5) (19)

- 0.5 mg/day for children <5 years old

- 1.0 mg/day for children 5 to 10 years old

- 1.5 mg/day for children >10 years old

- A maximum dose of 3mg/d in adults

The severity and outcome of colchicine intoxication are directly related to the dose ingested. The lethal dose begins for doses below 0.5mg/kg. It has already been reported that minor toxicity with only gastrointestinal symptomatology can occur at doses <0.5mg/kg, 0.5 to 0.8mg/kg results in major toxicity (multivisceral failure with bone marrow aplasia), and oral doses >0.8mg/kg can be fatal. (20) (21) (22)

Our patient ingested a dose of 1 mg/kg/d, i.e. higher than the supposed lethal dose.

There is no screening technique or colchicine assay that can be used in an emergency. Several analytical techniques have been developed, but the time required to deliver results is inadequate for emergency situations. (19)

In our case, we received the colchicinemia results 3 days after plasma sampling.

Plasma and urine colchicine can be determined by radioimmunoassay,(23) by gas chromatography coupled to a mass spectrometer,(24) high-pressure liquid chromatography coupled to a diode array detector or a tandem mass spectrometer. (25) (26)

We used the high-pressure liquid chromatography assay technique available at the urgent medical assistance center in Tunis.

In fact, although the mortality rate is correlated more with the presumed dose ingested than with plasma concentration, plasma dosage is still necessary to formally confirm intoxication and allow better interpretation of the clinical complications observed during follow-up. (26)

In view of the erratic diagnosis, our patient's colchicinemia level was measured on D9 after ingestion, and came back at 9 mg/ml, thus exceeding the therapeutic range.

This first measurement does not reflect the peak because the T max could not be determined due to delayed medical management. As colchicine is rapidly absorbed through the gastrointestinal mucosa, peak plasma levels are usually measured between 0.5 and 3 hours after oral administration. (8) (27)

This single dose of colchicine remained detectable in the blood even at D13. However, the plasma dosage was quantified at < 7mg/ml, i.e. below the toxic dose.

3. Toxidromes:

3.a: clinical manifestations:

Three phases of colchicine intoxication have been described in the literature. (28)

***1 phase:**

 -digestive problems:

The first phase of colchicine intoxication is characteristic of the first 24 hours, and is dominated by gastrointestinal symptoms such as nausea, vomiting, diarrhea and abdominal pain. (21) (22)

 The same symptomatology was observed in our patient on D1.

-hemorrhagic manifestations:

The literature describes the occurrence of melena during this phase.(29) (30) This symptom was not found in our patient.

-hemodynamic disorders:

Hypotension due to hypovolemia has also been reported in cases of colchicine intoxication as early as the first phase.(31) On admission, our patient presented with an initial blood pressure of 80/60 mm Hg.

***The second phase:**

This is the most critical phase, occurring between 24 hours and 7 days after intake, and corresponds to multi-visceral failure. (20)

At this stage, sudden death can occur as a result of acute respiratory failure. On the other hand, the main cause of death is heart failure such as rhythm disorders, atrioventricular block, myocardial depression, ventricular fibrillation or myocarditis.(28) (31) (32)

Neurological disorders have also been described, including confusion, hallucinations, convulsions, coma and sensory and motor disturbances. (28) (33)

During this period, weight gain due to interstitial edema has been described.

In this case, neurological disturbances such as confusion and hallucination were observed as early as D6. On the other hand, no cardiorespiratory failure or cardiac rhythm disturbance was observed in our patient. Weight gain was absent in our observation.

However, previously unreported cheilitis appeared in our patient at D6.

***3 phase:**

In two to three weeks' time, the third phase appears: the organ resolution and recovery phase, associated with the appearance of transient alopecia, neuromyopathy and weight loss. (32) (33) (34)

This last phase was observed in our case with the appearance of alopecia at D10.

3.b: biological manifestations:

*** 1 phase:**

Hyperleukocytosis has been reported within the first 24 hours. (20) (35)

In our case, leukocytes were 10300 el/mm3 on Day 1.

***2 phase:**

The second phase appears between days 2 and 7 and is characterized by a drop in coagulation factors. Medullar aplasia appears abruptly from day 3 onwards. Liver failure, renal failure and rhabdomyolysis have also been reported in this phase. During this period, there is water leakage into the interstitial sector (through alteration of capillary endothelial membranes), accompanied by hyponatremia. Other ionic disorders have also been observed: hypokalemia, hypocalcemia and hypophosphatemia. Colchicine intoxication gives rise to metabolic acidosis or lactic acidosis. (35) (36) (37)

Our patient successively presented these biological disorders. She developed renal and hepatic failure and rhabdomyolysis on D1; ionic disorders (hyponatremia as early as H24, hypocalcemia on D4 and hypokalemia on D7); and serious hematological complications as early as D4 (pancytopenia).

***3 phase:**

The third phase of colchicine intoxication occurs only in cases with a favorable evolution. It is characterized by reactive hyperleukocytosis. (37)

Rebound hyperleukocytosis was observed in our patient at D8.

4. literature review:

Acute colchicine intoxication is rare and potentially serious. We conducted a literature review of cases of pediatric colchicine intoxication. Our research collated 42 sporadic cases of colchicine intoxication between 1981 and 2021.

4-1: Breakdown of poisoning by year

The highest number of cases of colchicine poisoning occurred in 2016 (nine cases). Seven cases were reported in 2011 and 2009.

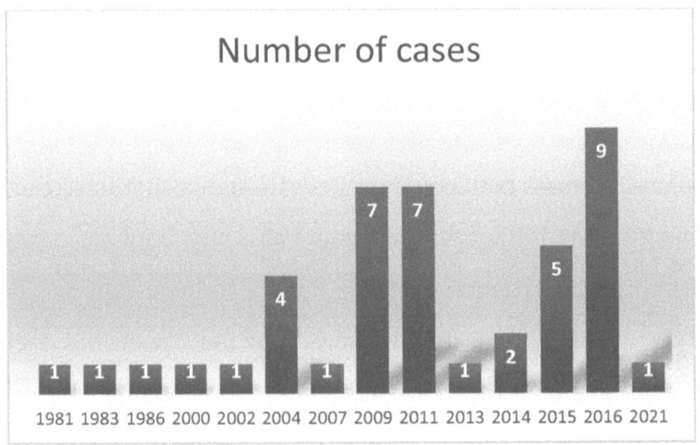

Figure 3: Distribution of colchicine poisoning cases by year

4-2: Breakdown of intoxication by age

The age of intoxication ranged from 1 to 16 years. The age group most affected was between 1 and 5 years.

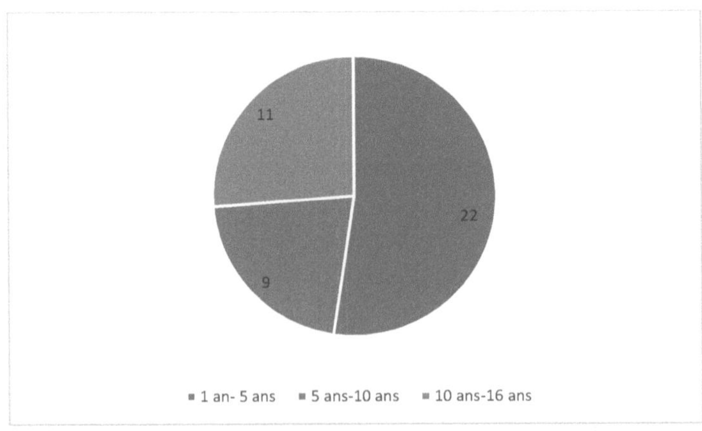

Figure4: Distribution of intoxication according to age

4-3: Circumstances of intoxication

Colchicine intoxication was accidental in 23 cases. It was secondary to a suicide attempt in 10 cases.

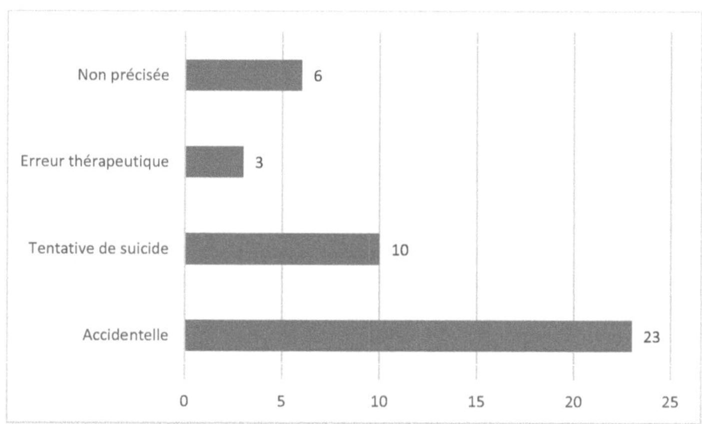

Figure 5: Circumstances of colchicine intoxication

4-4 Toxidromes:

In this review of the literature, the three clinico-biological phases previously described following colchicine intoxication were described in all observations. Digestive symptomatology in the foreground, followed by multivisceral failure.

4-5 Toxicological analysis

Determination of colchicinemia and presumed ingested dose is the main prognostic element in colchicine intoxication. Ten patients out of 42 observations exceeded the lethal dose of 0.8 mg/kg, of whom only 4 survived. Thirty patients ingested a dose of colchicine lower than 0.8 mg/kg, 26 of whom had a favorable outcome.

A review of the literature on the diagnostic, therapeutic and evolutionary aspects of colchicine intoxication is presented in Table II.

Date	Author	Age	Type of poisoning	ISD	Clinical manifestations	Biological manifestations	Treatment	Evolution
1981	Stapczynski et al. (38)	16 years old	Unknown	12 mg (0.26mg/kg)	Vomiting diarrhea tachycardia tachypnea	Hypokalemia 2.7 mEq/L, hyperleukocytosis 25300/mm3	Gastric lavage, perfusion, correction of hypokalemia, oxygen therapy.	Deaths
1983	Murray et al. (39)	15 years	Unknown	24 mg (0.5mg/kg)	Cardiac, digestive and respiratory complications.	Hematological complications.	Not mentioned.	Survival.
1986	Hobson C.H and Rankin, A. (40)	15 years	Suicide attempt	18 mg (0.45mg/kg)	Vomiting diarrhea melena dehydration Tachycardia, hypotension, Tachypnea, hypoxemia, ECG signs of myocardial ischemia	hyperleukocytosis to 39700/mm3, coagulation disorder	Perfusion, oesotracheal intubation, vitamin K, dopamine, epinephrine	Death.
2000	Goldbart, A. et al. (41)	8 years old	Treated for FMF	Unknown	Vomiting, diarrhea, melena, tachypnea, hypoxemia, tachycardia, fever, hypotension, LVEF 21%. Alopecia at D8.	Pancytopenia, hepatic cytolysis, hyponatremia, accelerated SV, rebound hyperleukocytosis at D 10.	Perfusion, antibiotic therapy, oesotracheal intubation, vasoactive drugs, vitamin K, FFP transfusion, 1 RGC, 1 platelet pellet.	Survival.
2002	Guven, A.G et al. (42)	4 years	Accidental	1.3 - 1.5 mg (0.1mg/kg)	Abdominal pain, diarrhea, vomiting, melena, ecchymosis, petechiae, confusion, arterial hypotension, tachycardia, tachypnea, enanthema of the buccal	Pancytopenia, hypokalemia, hepatic cytolysis	Not specified	Survival.

2004	Atas, B. et al.(43)	12 years	Not mentioned	3 mg (0.12mg/kg)	mucosa, erythema nodosum lower limbs, bullous erythema of the trunk and extremities, alopecia at D6. Coma glascow: 06/15 , tachycardia, tachypnea, arterial hypotension, ROT abolished.	Anemia, hyperleukocytosis to 48000/mm3, hypocalcemia to 1.65 mmol/L, metabolic acidosis, hepatic cytolysis.	Symptomatic treatment, gastric lavage, oesotracheal intubation.	Death.
2004	Atas, B. et al.(43)	02 years old	Accidental	6 mg (0.5mg /kg)	Vomiting, supraventricular tachycardia, tachypnea, arterial hypotension, alopecia at D7.	Anemia, hyperleukocytosis to 25600/mm3, severe thrombocytopenia to 10000/mm3, hypocalcemia to 1.77 mmol/L, hepatic cytolysis, rhabdomyolysis, rebound hyperleukocytosis at D7.	Gastric lavage, activated charcoal, infusion and correction of hypocalcemia, antibiotic therapy.	Survival.
2004	Atas, B. et al.(43)	27 months	Accidental	10 mg (0.83mg/kg)	Coma Glasgow 05/15, vomiting, diarrhea, tachycardia, tachypnea, arterial hypotension, hepatomegaly, ROT abolished.	Hyperleukocytosis to 55100/mm3, hypocalcemia to 1.8 mmol/L, hyperuricemia, hepatic cytolysis, metabolic acidosis.	Perfusion, gastric lavage, activated charcoal.	Death.

2004	Atas, B. et al.(43)	3.5 years	Accidental	25 mg (1.5mg /kg)	Tachycardia, tachypnea, the rest of the examination is strictly normal.	No biological abnormalities.	Gastric lavage, activated charcoal.	Survival.
2007	Suat Bic,er, MD. et al. (44)	3 years	Not mentioned	0.7 mg/Kg	Vomiting, fever, diarrhea, tachycardia, tachypnea, arterial hypotension, ROT abolished, GCS 13, cerebral edema, convulsion, alopecia at D14.	Renal failure, hyponatremia, pancytopenia, rebound hyperleukocytosis at D6, DIC, hyperuricemia, hypocalcemia.	Perfusion, antibiotic therapy, dobutamine, furosemide, transfusion of FFP RGCs and platelets, Prazosin, captopril, Phenytoin.	Survival.
2009	Karacan M , et al. (45)	4 years	Accidental	0.5 mg (0.03mg/kg)	Vomiting.	Hyperleukocytosis, hepatic cytolysis, rhabdomyolysis.	Gastric lavage, activated charcoal, vitamin K.	Survival
2009	Karacan M, et al.(45)	4 years	Not specified	0.33 mg/Kg	Asymptomatic.	No abnormalities.	Gastric lavage, activated charcoal.	Survival.
2009	Karacan M, et al.(45)	5 years	Accidental	Not specified	Fever, vomiting, drowsiness, tachycardia, tachypnea, cyanosis, hypotension, heart failure.	Hepatic cytolysis, renal failure, rhabdomyolysis, ionic disorders.	Gastric lavage, activated charcoal, vasoactive drugs.	Death.
2009	Karacan M. et al.(45)	9 years old	Suicide attempt.	15 mg (0.85mg/kg)	Asymptomatic.	No abnormalities.	Gastric lavage, activated charcoal.	Survival
2009	Karacan M. et al.(45)	1 year	Not specified.	1.5 mg (0.15mg/kg)	Vomiting.	No abnormalities.	Abstention	Survival
2009	Karacan M. et al.(45)	2.5 years	Accidental.	3.5 mg (0.29mg/kg)	Asymptomatic.	Hepatic cytolysis.	Gastric lavage, activated charcoal.	Survival
2009	Karacan M. et al.(45)	3.5 years	Accidental.	5 mg (0.33mg/kg)	Vomiting, asthenia.	Hyperleukocytosis, hepatic cytolysis, rhabdomyolysis.	Gastric lavage, activated charcoal.	Survival

2011	Ozdemir R. et al.(46)	3 years	Accidental.	0.5 mg/ Kg	Vomiting.	No abnormalities.	Gastric lavage, activated charcoal.	Survival.
2011	Ozdemir R. et al.(46)	3 years	Accidental.	0.6 mg/Kg	Asymptomatic.	Hepatic cytolysis.	Gastric lavage, activated charcoal.	Survival.
2011	Ozdemir R. et al.(46)	3 years	Accidental.	1.1 mg/Kg	Vomiting.	Hyperleukocytosis.	Gastric lavage, activated charcoal, hemodialysis, plasma exchange, vasoactive drugs.	Survival.
2011	Ozdemir R. et al.(46)	5 years	Accidental.	1.25 mg/Kg	Vomiting, asthenia.	Pancytopenia, hepatic cytolysis, renal failure, rhabdomyolysis.	Activated charcoal, hemodialysis, plasma exchange, vasoactive drugs, granulocyte colony-stimulating factor.	Death.
2011	Ozdemir R. et al.(46)	14 years old	Suicide attempt	0.5 mg/Kg	Vomiting.	Hyperleukocytosis, hepatic cytolysis, rhabdomyolysis, renal failure.	Activated charcoal, hemodialysis, intra-aortic counterpulsation balloon.	Death.
2011	Ozdemir R. et al.(46)	14 years old	Suicide attempt	0.9 mg/ Kg	Asymptomatic.	Pancytopenia.	Gastric lavage, activated charcoal, plasma exchange, granulocyte colony-stimulating factor.	Survival.
2011	Ozdemir R. et al.(46)	16 years old	Suicide attempt	1.4 mg/Kg	Vomiting, diarrhea.	Hyperleukocytosis, rhabdomyolysis, renal	Gastric lavage, activated charcoal,	Death.

2013	Wasser scheid, K. et al. (47)	14 years old	Suicide attempt	12.5 mg (0.35mg/kg)	Nausea, abdominal pain.	Low TP at 48%.	Activated charcoal, sodium sulfate, vitamin K, infusion.	Survival.
						failure, hepatic cytolysis.	extracorporeal membrane oxygenation (ECMO).	
2014	Suar C. Kilic, et al.(48)	3 years	accidental	0.2 mg/Kg	Vomiting, disturbed consciousness, fever, tachycardia, hypotension, tachypnea, petechiae, hepatosplenomegaly.	Hyperleukocytosis at Day 1, hepatic cytolysis, renal failure, hyperuricemia, ionic disorders, rhabdomyolysis, pancytopenia at Day 3, rebound hyperleukocytosis at Day 6, elevated D-dimer, blood culture positive for staphylococcus aureus at Day 2.	Adequate hydration, allopurinol, electrolyte correction, antibiotic therapy, FFP and platelet transfusion, granulocyte colony-stimulating factor.	Survival.
2014	Malbora B. et al.(49)	9 years old	Accidental.	15 mg. (0.5mg/kg)	Vomiting, diarrhea, fever, hepatomegaly, splenomegaly, arterial hypotension, BAV.	Thrombocytopenia, hepatic cytolysis, hyperferritinemia, renal failure, hyperkalemia, rhabdomyolysis.	Plasma exchange, vitamin K, FFP transfusion.	Death.
2015	Kintz, P. et al.(50)	4 years	Therapeutic error.	8mg on two consecutive days. (1.14mg/kg)	Vomiting, diarrhea, pericarditis.	Multivisceral failure, colchicinemia 14.7 ng/ml.	Not specified.	Death.

2015	Kisaars lan. P et al.(51)	3.5 years	Accide ntal.	8 mg. (0.82m g/kg)	Tachycardia.	Hyperleukoc ytosis, hepatic cytolysis, rhabdomyol ysis.	Gastric lavage, activated charcoal, plasma exchange	Death.
2015	Kisaars lan. P et al.(51)	5 years	Accide ntal	1 mg (0.05m g/kg)	Vomiting, diarrhea, fever, alopecia.	Leukopenia, rebound hyperleukoc ytosis, hepatic cytolysis, hyponatremia.	Symptomati c treatment.	Survival.
2015	Kisaars lan. P et al.(51)	15 years	Suicide attempt .	10 mg. (0.22m g/kg)	Fever, abdominal pain, vomiting, alopecia.	Pancytopeni a, rebound hyperleukoc ytosis, renal failure, metabolic acidosis.	Symptomati c treatment,	Survival.
2015	Kisaars lan. P et al.(51)	15 years	Suicide attempt .	5 mg. (0.11m g/kg)	Asymptomatic.	No abnormalities.	Gastric lavage.	Survival.
2016	Polat, E. et al.(52)	1.5 years	acciden tal	0.16 mg/kg	Asymptomatic.	Hyperleukoc ytosis, rhabdomyol ysis.	Gastric lavage, activated charcoal.	Survival.
2016	Polat, E. et al.(52)	2 years	Accide ntal.	0.3 mg/Kg	Asymptomatic.	Hyperleukoc ytosis.	Gastric lavage, activated charcoal.	Survival.
2016	Polat, E. et al.(52)	4 years	Accide ntal.	0.6 mg/Kg	Asymptomatic.	Hyperleukoc ytosis.	Gastric lavage, activated charcoal.	Survival.
2016	Polat, E. et al.(52)	4 years	Accide ntal.	0.11 mg/Kg	Asymptomatic.	No abnormalities.	Gastric lavage, activated charcoal.	Survival.
2016	Polat, E. et al.	4.5 years	Accide ntal	0.6 mg/Kg	Vomiting	No abnormalities	Gastric lavage, activated charcoal	survival
2016	Polat, E. et al.(52)	8 years old	Accide ntal	0.52 mg/Kg	Vomiting, nausea, diarrhea.	Hyperleukoc ytosis, hepatic cytolysis, rhabdomyol ysis.	External pacemaker, vasoactive drugs, antiarrhyth mic (unspecified).	Death.

2016	Polat, E. et al.(52)	8.5 years	Suicide attempt.	0.5 mg/Kg	Vomiting, nausea, diarrhea.	Leukopenia, thrombocytopenia, hepatic cytolysis, rhabdomyolysis.	External pacemaker, plasma exchange, vasoactive drugs.	Death.
2016	Polat, E. et al.(52)	10 years	Accidental.	0.12 mg/Kg	Nausea, vomiting.	ASAT slightly elevated.	Gastric lavage, activated charcoal.	Survival.
2016	Polat, E. et al.(52)	16 years old	Suicide attempt.	0.84 mg/Kg.	Nausea, vomiting, diarrhea.	Hyperleukocytosis, hepatic cytolysis, rhabdomyolysis.	Plasma exchange, vasoactive drugs.	Death.
2021	Pérez Marín M. et al.(53)	4 years	Therapeutic error.	7 mg. (0.53mg/kg)	Vomiting, diarrhea, tachycardia, tachypnea, hypotension, somnolence, hypoxemia, congestive heart failure, anuria, polyneuromyopathy, alopecia at D19.	Renal failure, hepatic cytolysis, hyperbilirubinemia, hyperleukocytosis on Day 1, leukopenia on Day 3, thrombocytopenia, colchicinemia 0.2µg/L on Day 16.	Activated charcoal, tracheal intubation, non-invasive ventilation, vasoactive drugs, antibiotic therapy, ECMO, hemodialysis, FFP and platelet transfusion, granulocyte colony-stimulating factor, physiotherapy.	Survival.

5. Processing:

The main treatment for colchicine intoxication remains symptomatic, in the absence of specific therapy. (20)

At present, the literature does not provide a specific antidote for colchicine intoxication. In fact, gastric lavage followed by passage of activated charcoal is crucial within 60 minutes of ingestion to limit the enterohepatic cycle. (54)

This evacuation treatment was not carried out in this particular case, given the delay in taking charge.

In the literature, a study by Ozdemir et al. demonstrated the benefit of plasma exchange in colchicine elimination and its contribution to the treatment of multivisceral failure. (46) (55)

In some cases of colchicine intoxication, dialysis purification has been described at less than 5%. Hemodialysis, like plasmapheresis, does not eliminate colchicine due to its large volume of distribution and high protein binding. It is, however, useful in cases of acute renal failure. (56) (57)

Our patient developed acute functional renal failure, which was controlled by symptomatic treatment within the first few hours of care.

Prompt symptomatic treatment is essential to ensure a better prognosis. (46) (55) (58)

In our patient, only symptomatic treatments (vasopressor drugs, antibiotic therapy, hydroelectric rebalancing, correction of the acid-base balance, platelet transfusion, administration of vit K, etc.) were administered in the ICU, enabling the successive organ failures and complications to be corrected.

Immunotherapy with specific anti-colchicine Fab antibodies may be effective in colchicine intoxication. To date, this therapy is only available on an experimental basis, despite encouraging results from animal and human experimental data. (46) (59)

This alternative is not available in our country.

In the case presented here, the initial administration of IV immunoglobulin in the face of the diagnostic hypothesis of MIS-C, could contribute to the favorable evolution.

6. F prognostic actors:

Various studies have proposed the objective of identifying prognostic factors and progression to death for patients with colchicine intoxication.

The presumed ingested dose (DSI) is a consistently highlighted prognostic factor. The clinical picture and mortality rate appear to be closely linked to the dose ingested.

If the dose absorbed is less than 0.5 mg/kg, intoxication manifests itself as more or less intense digestive disorders, and purely biological blood disorders. After a dose of between 0.5 and 0.8 mg/kg of body weight, the digestive disorders and haemostasis disturbances are identical, but the evolution is towards bone marrow aplasia. Mortality rate > 10%, due either to hemorrhage or uncontrolled sepsis.

At doses equal to or greater than 0.8 mg/kg, initial digestive disturbances with consumption of coagulation factors are rapidly accompanied by cardiovascular collapse with a component of acute cardiac failure, with a mortality rate of 100%. (19) (60)

In our patient's case, the DSI was 1mg/Kg, with a possibly unfavorable outcome according to the literature.

Prognostic assessment must also take into account the biological effects of this ingested dose, which seem best illustrated by early hyperleukocytosis (greater than 15,000/mm3) and a fall in the prothrombin level to below 20% within the first 24 hours.(19)

In the present case, the first 24 hours' work-up showed a white blood cell count of 10500 el/mm3 with a prothrombin level of 51%, which suggests a reassuring evolution.

The risk of colchicine accumulation in the event of liver damage also plays an important role. Several factors are likely to affect colchicine's hepatic clearance, such as changes in the liver's purification activity, as seen in certain pathologies such as primary biliary cirrhosis or hepatic cirrhosis, or associated treatments, mainly CYP3A4 and P-gp inhibitors. Plasma concentrations of colchicine metabolites are less than 5% of those of the parent compound.(60) (61)

In the present case, no drugs metabolized via CYP3A or P-gp competitors were found.

The occurrence of adverse reactions in patients with renal impairment shows that changes in renal clearance of colchicine represent a risk factor. In patients with renal impairment, the risk of accumulation appears to become significant at creatinine clearances of less than 50 ml/min. Indeed, the elimination half-life of colchicine can be four times longer in patients with major renal impairment.(60) (62)

Rapid improvement in renal clearance with symptomatic treatment contributed to our patient's favorable outcome.

Conclusion:

This case illustrates a severe pediatric intoxication with colchicine in a 13-year-old girl, with suicidal intent. The initial clinico-biological picture was not very specific, and the intoxication was not announced at the start of treatment, leading to a misdiagnosis. On the other hand, adequate management of the various organ failures, even in the absence of a precise etiological diagnosis, led to a favorable outcome. There is no antidote to colchicine. Treatment was symptomatic only.

Our review of the literature revealed the following points:

1- Pediatric cases of colchicine intoxication were described in 42 different observations between 1981 and 2021, with ages ranging from 1 to 16 years.

2- The clinical and biological manifestations of colchicine intoxication pass through three successive phases:

The first phase is characteristic of the first 24 hours and is manifested by digestive and hemorrhagic symptoms, hemodynamic disorders and hyperleukocytosis.

The second phase takes place between 24 hours and 7 days after intake, and corresponds to multi-visceral failure, associated with neurological disorders. Medullar aplasia and a drop in coagulation factors may also occur during this phase.

The final phase, the resolution phase, occurs after two to three weeks and is characterized by organ recovery and the appearance of transient alopecia. Reactive hyperleukocytosis may be observed during this phase.

3- Treatment of colchicine intoxication is essentially symptomatic, to deal with various organ failures. To this day, there is no specific antidote for colchicine.

4- The prognosis, according to the various studies consulted, showed a close relationship between the dose of DSI ingested and the mortality rate.

In fact, a dose of 0.5 mg/kg causes more or less intense digestive problems, with blood crase disorders of a purely biological nature.

A dose of between 0.5 and 0.8 mg/kg, in addition to causing digestive problems, can also lead to bone marrow aplasia. Hemorrhage in this case is responsible for a mortality rate of over 10%. Studies have also shown that a dose equal to or greater than 0.8 mg/kg is rapidly accompanied by cardiovascular collapse with a component of acute cardiac failure, with a mortality rate of 100%.

Other prognostic factors also influence the outcome of patients suffering from colchicine intoxication. These include early hyperleukocytosis (above 15,000/mm^3) and a fall in prothrombin levels below 20% within the first 24 hours, the onset of liver failure and renal failure.

In the present case, our patient benefited from rapid and adequate management despite the absence of an initial diagnostic orientation towards intoxication, which led to a favorable outcome despite an ISD greater than 0.8mg/kg; a dose assumed to be lethal.

At the end of this dissertation we propose to:

- Set up a national register of drug poisoning by pharmacovigilance centers, in collaboration with pediatric departments and pediatric intensive care units, for epidemiological purposes.

- Provide a personal leaflet for patients treated with colchicine (in Arabic and French) containing the prescribed dose, any drug interactions and the first clinical signs of overdose that should prompt immediate consultation, stressing the importance of understanding the dosage schedule and the dangers of taking colchicine without medical advice.

- Promote research in immunology laboratories with a view to introducing specific anti-colchicine immunotherapy, which appears to be a therapeutic option for the future, since today, despite advances in resuscitation, severe forms of colchicine overdose are still in most cases refractory to available measures.

References

1.   Chappey O, Scherrmann J. Colchicine: recent data on its pharmacokinetics and clinical pharmacology. Rev Médecine Interne. Oct 1995;16(10):782-9.

2.   Miyachi Y, Taniguchi S, Ozaki M, Horio T. Colchicine in the treatment of the cutaneous manifestations of Behcet's disease. Br J Dermatol. Jan 1981;104(1):67-70.

3.   Bhat A, Naguwa SM, Cheema GS, Gershwin ME. Colchicine Revisited. Ann N Y Acad Sci. Sept 2009;1173(1):766-73.

4.   Graening T, Schmalz HG. Total Syntheses of Colchicine in Comparison: A Journey through 50 Years of Synthetic Organic Chemistry. Angew Chem Int Ed. June 21, 2004;43(25):3230-56.

5.   Knieper AM, Klotsche J, Föll D, Wittkowski H, Lainka E, Kallinich T. Colchicine therapy in children with FMF. Pediatr Rheumatol. Dec 2015;13(S1):O44.

6.   Putterman C, Ben-Chetrit E, Caraco Y, Levy M. Colchicine intoxication: Clinical pharmacology, risk factors, features, and management. Semin Arthritis Rheum. Dec 1991;21(3):143-55.

7.   Sapra S, Bhalla Y, Nandani, Sharma S, Singh G, Nepali K, et al. Colchicine and its various physicochemical and biological aspects. Med Chem Res. Feb 2013;22(2):531-47.

8.   Rochdi M, Sabouraud A, Girre C, Venet R, Scherrmann JM. Pharmacokinetics and absolute bioavailability of colchicine after i. v. and oral administration in healthy human volunteers and elderly subjects. Eur J Clin Pharmacol [Internet]. 1994 [cited March 14, 2022];46(4). Available from: http://link.springer.com/10.1007/BF00194404

9.   Amoura Z, Schermann JM, Zerah X, Wechsler B, Godeau P. First evidence of transplacental passage of colchicine during periodic illness. Rev Médecine Interne. June 1993;14(6):593.

10.   Slobodnick A, Shah B, Pillinger MH, Krasnokutsky S. Colchicine: Old and New. Am J Med. May 2015;128(5):461-70.

11.   Speeg KV, Maldonado AL, Liaci J, Muirhead D. Effect of cyclosporine on colchicine secretion by a liver canalicular transporter studiedin vivo. Hepatology. May 1992;15(5):899-903.

12.   Lidar M. Colchicine nonresponsiveness in familial mediterranean fever: clinical, genetic, pharmacokinetic, and socioeconomic characterization. Semin Arthritis Rheum. Feb 2004;33(4):273-82.

13.   Niel E, Scherrmann JM. Colchicine today. Joint Bone Spine. Dec 2006;73(6):672-8.

14.   Cronstein BN, Molad Y, Reibman J, Balakhane E, Levin RI, Weissmann G. Colchicine alters the quantitative and qualitative display of selectins on endothelial cells and neutrophils. J Clin Invest. August 1, 1995;96(2):994-1002.

15.   Matsumura N, Mizushima Y. Leukocyte movement and colchicine treatment in Behcet's disease. The Lancet. Oct 1975;306(7939):813.

16.   Leung YY, Yao Hui LL, Kraus VB. Colchicine-Update on mechanisms of action and therapeutic uses. Semin Arthritis Rheum. Dec 2015;45(3):341-50.

17.   Lu Y, Chen Y, Kao Y, Lin Y, Yeh Y, Chen S, et al. Colchicine modulates calcium homeostasis and electrical property of HL-1 cells. J Cell Mol Med. June 2016;20(6):1182-90.

18. Ehrenfeld M, Levy M, Margalioth EJ, Eliakim M. The Effects of Long-term Colchicine Therapy on Male Fertility in Patients with Familial Mediterranean Fever. Andrologia. 24 Apr 2009;18(4):420-6.

19. Wolf A, Oliver M, Nau A, Boulliat C, Puidupin A, Peytel E, et al. A case of lethal colchicine intoxication. Ann Biol Clin (Paris). Sept 2009;67(5):581-5.

20. Picard W, Julliac B, Morel N, Sztark F, Dabadie P. Fatal multivisceral failure presumably induced by chronic colchicine overdose. J Eur Urgences. March 2007;20(1):7-10.

21. Finkelstein Y, Aks SE, Hutson JR, Juurlink DN, Nguyen P, Dubnov-Raz G, et al. Colchicine poisoning: the dark side of an ancient drug. Clin Toxicol. June 2010;48(5):407-14.

22. Gunasekaran K, Mathew DE, Sudarsan TI, Iyyadurai R. Fatal colchicine intoxication by ingestion of *Gloriosa superba* tubers. BMJ Case Rep. May 16, 2019;12(5):e228718.

23. Scherrmann JM, Boudet L, Pontikis R, Hoang-Nam N, Fournier E. A sensitive radioimmunoassay for colchicine. J Pharm Pharmacol. Apr 12, 2011;32(1):800-2.

24. Vollmer AC, Wagmann L, Meyer MR. Toxic plants-Detection of colchicine in a fast systematic clinical toxicology screening using liquid chromatography-mass spectrometry. Drug Test Anal. Feb 2022;14(2):377-81.

25. Cheze M, Deveaux M, Pepin G. Liquid Chromatography-Tandem Mass Spectrometry for the Determination of Colchicine in Postmortem Body Fluids. Case Report of Two Fatalities and Review of the Literature. J Anal Toxicol. 1 Oct 2006;30(8):593-8.

26.   Abe E, Lemaire-Hurtel AS, Duverneuil C, Etting I, Guillot E, de Mazancourt P, et al. A Novel LC-ESI-MS-MS Method for Sensitive Quantification of Colchicine in Human Plasma: Application to Two Case Reports. J Anal Toxicol. 1 Apr 2006;30(3):210-5.

27.   Rochdi M, Sabouraud A, Baud FJ, Bismuth C, Scherrmann JM. Toxicokinetics of Colchicine in Humans: Analysis of Tissue, Plasma and Urine Data in Ten Cases. Hum Exp Toxicol. Nov 1992;11(6):510-6.

28.   Folpini A, Furfori P. Colchicine Toxicity Clinical Features and Treatment. Massive Overdose Case Report. J Toxicol Clin Toxicol. Jan 1995;33(1):71-7.

29.   Cerquaglia C, Diaco M, Nucera G, Regina M, Montalto M, Manna R. Pharmacological and Clinical Basis of Treatment of Familial Mediterranean Fever (FMF) with Colchicine or Analogues: An Update. Curr Drug Target - Inflamm Allergy. 1 Feb 2005;4(1):117-24.

30.   Watanabe-Kusunoki K, Kato M, Oki Y, Shimizu T, Kusunoki Y, Furukawa S, et al. Parallel disease activity of Behçet's disease with renal and entero involvements: a case report. BMC Nephrol. Dec 2021;22(1):122.

31.   Sauder Ph, Kopferschmitt J, Jaeger A, Mantz JM. Haemodynamic Studies in Eight Cases of Acute Colchicine Poisoning. Hum Toxicol. Apr 1983;2(2):169-73.

32.   Maxwell MJ. Accidental colchicine overdose. A case report and literature review. Emerg Med J. May 1, 2002;19(3):265-6.

33.   Carr AA. Colchicine Toxicity. Arch Intern Med. 1 Jan 1965;115(1):29.

34.   Kuncl RW, Duncan G, Watson D, Alderson K, Rogawski MA, Peper M. Colchicine Myopathy and Neuropathy. N Engl J Med. June 18, 1987;316(25):1562-8.

35.   Dixon WE, Malden W. Colchicine with special reference to its mode of action and effect on bone-marrow. J Physiol. May 6, 1908;37(1):50-76.

36.   Huang WH, Hsu CW, Yu CC. Colchicine Overdose-Induced Acute Renal Failure and Electrolyte Imbalance. Ren Fail. 1 Jan 2007;29(3):367-70.

37.   Altman A, Szyper-Kravitz M, Shoenfeld Y. Colchicine-induced rhabdomyolysis. Clin Rheumatol. Dec 2007;26(12):2197-9.

38.   Stapczynski JS, Rothstein RJ, Gaye WA, Niemann JT. Colchicine overdose: Report of two cases and review of the literature. Ann Emerg Med. Jul 1981;10(7):364-9.

39.   Ss M, Kg K, Jc M, Dn M. Acute toxicity after excessive ingestion of colchicine. undefined [Internet]. 1983 [cited March 16, 2022]; Available from: https://www.semanticscholar.org/paper/Acute-toxicity-after-excessive-ingestion-of-Ss-Kg/4e23529633e879880fb2d917cd20d0629f3e4f6a

40.   Hobson CH, Rankin APN. A fatal colchicine overdose. Anaesth Intensive Care. Nov 1986;14(4):453-5.

41.   Goldbart A, Press J, Sofer S, Kapelushnik J. Near fatal acute colchicine intoxication in a child. A case report. Eur J Pediatr. 20 nov 2000;159(12):895-7.

42.   Güven AG, Bahat E, Akman S, Artan R, Erol M. Late Diagnosis of Severe Colchicine Intoxication. Pediatrics. May 1, 2002;109(5):971-3.

43.   Ataş B, Çaksen H, Tuncer O, Kirimi E, Akgün C, Odabaş D. Four children with colchicine poisoning. Hum Exp Toxicol. Jul 2004;23(7):353-6.

44.   Bi??er S, Soysal DD, ??tak A, ????sel R, Karab??c??o??lu M, Uzel N. Acute Colchicine Intoxication in a Child: A Case Report. Pediatr Emerg Care. May 2007;23(5):314-7.

45.   Karacan M, Olgun H, Yildirim ZK, Karakelleoğlu C, Ceviz N. Colchicine Poisoning in Children: 7 Case Reports. Güncel Pediatri. Dec 1, 2009;7(3):96-100.

46.   Ozdemir R, Bayrakci B, Teksam O. Fatal poisoning in children: Acute Colchicine intoxication and new treatment approaches. Clin Toxicol. Oct 2011;49(8):739-43.

47.   Wasserscheid K, Backendorf A, Michna D, Mallmann R, Hoffmann B. Long-term Outcome After Suicidal Colchicine Intoxication in a 14-Year-Old Girl: Case Report and Review of Literature. Pediatr Emerg Care. Jan 2013;29(1):89-92.

48.   Kilic SC, Alaygut D, Unal E, Koç E, Patiroglu T. Acute Colchicine Intoxication Complicated With Extramedullary Hematopoiesis Due to Filgrastim in a Child. J Pediatr Hematol Oncol. oct 2014;36(7):e460-2.

49.   Malbora B, Polat E, Akyuz SG. Hemophagocytic Lymphohistiocytosis and Pelger-Huët Anomaly Associated with Colchicine Intoxication. Hematol Rep. June 19, 2014;6(2):5356.

50.   Kintz P, Jamey C, Martrille L, Raul JS. Colchicine and pediatric intoxication: about an accidental death and review of the literature. Toxicol Anal Clin. March 2016;28(1):79-84.

51.   Kisaarslan AP, Yel S, Yilmaz K, Akyildiz BN, Düşünsel R, Gündüz Z, et al. Colchicine Intoxication in Children: Four Case Reports. Arch Rheumatol. 2015;30(1):067-70.

52.   Polat E, Tuygun N, Akca H, Karacan CD. Evaluation of the Colchicine Poisoning Cases in a Pediatric Intensive Care Unit: Five Year Study. J Emerg Med. Apr 2017;52(4):499-503.

53.   Pérez Marín M, Prod'hom S, de Villiers SF, Ferry T, Amiet V, Natterer J, et al. Case Report: Colchicine Toxicokinetic Analysis in a Poisoned Child Requiring Extracorporeal Life Support. Front Pediatr. Apr 7, 2021;9:658347.

54.   Zawahir S, Gawarammana I, Dargan PI, Abdulghni M, Dawson AH. Activated charcoal significantly reduces the amount of colchicine released from *Gloriosa superba* in simulated gastric and intestinal media. Clin Toxicol. 14 Sep 2017;55(8):914-8.

55.   Demirkol D, Karacabey BN, Aygun F. Plasma Exchange Treatment in a Case of Colchicine Intoxication. Ther Apher Dial. Feb 2015;19(1):95-7.

56.   Kangin M, Talay MN, Tanriverdi Yilmaz S. Abstract P-106: PLASMAPHERESIS IN COLCHICINE POISONING. Pediatr Crit Care Med. June 2018;19:81.

57.   Simons RJ, Kingma DW. Fatal colchicine toxicity. Am J Med. March 1989;86(3):356-7.

58.   Hood RL. Colchicine poisoning. J Emerg Med. March 1994;12(2):171-7.

59.   Eddleston M, Persson H. Acute Plant Poisoning and Antitoxin Antibodies: Antivenoms. J Toxicol Clin Toxicol. Jan 2003;41(3):309-15.

60.   Allard M, Soichot M, Bourgogne E, Jaffal K, Megarbane B, Labat L. Colchicine intoxication: importance of initial management conditions. Toxicol Anal Clin. May 2019;31(2):S80.

61.   Leighton JA, Bay MK, Maldonado AL, Johnson RF, Schenker S, Speeg KV. The effect of liver dysfunction on colchicine pharmacokinetics in the rat. Hepatology. Feb 1990;11(2):210-5.

62.   Chappey ON, Niel E, Wautier JL, Hung PP, Dervichian M, Cattan D, et al. Colchicine disposition in human leukocytes after single and multiple oral administration. Clin Pharmacol Ther. Oct 1993;54(4):360-7.

CONTENTS

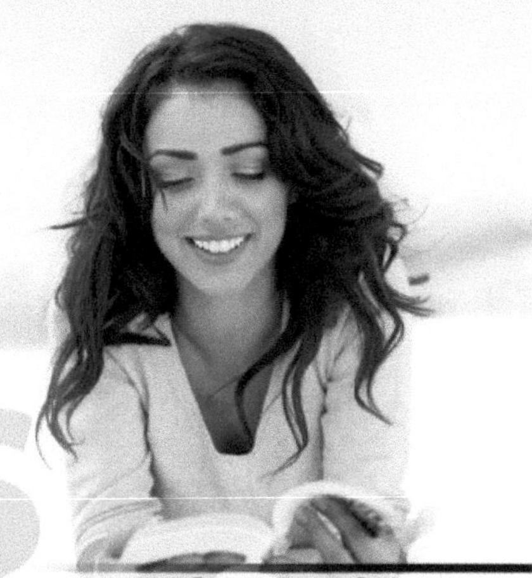

yes

I want morebooks!

Buy your books fast and straightforward online - at one of world's fastest growing online book stores! Environmentally sound due to Print-on-Demand technologies.

Buy your books online at
www.morebooks.shop

Kaufen Sie Ihre Bücher schnell und unkompliziert online – auf einer der am schnellsten wachsenden Buchhandelsplattformen weltweit! Dank Print-On-Demand umwelt- und ressourcenschonend produzi ert.

Bücher schneller online kaufen
www.morebooks.shop

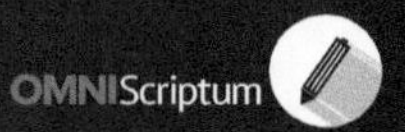

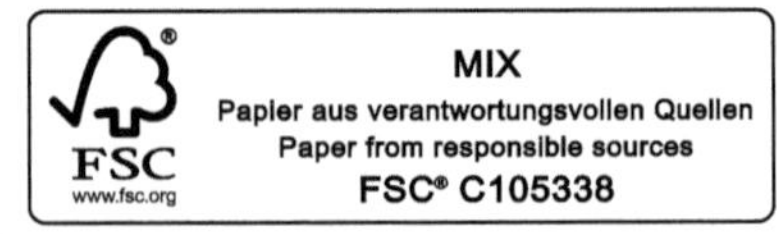

Printed by Books on Demand GmbH, Norderstedt / Germany